SIMPLE CHAIR YOGA FOR SENIORS OVER 60

Easy And Effective Seated Exercises Tailored For Individuals Over 60, Designed To Assist With Weight Loss And Enhance Balance.

Vanessa Meza

Table of Contents

INTRODUCTION TO CHAIR YOGA FOR SENIORS

A. Explanation of Chair Yoga:

Definition: Chair yoga is a modified form of yoga that can be done while sitting on a chair or using a chair for support. It incorporates gentle stretches, breathing exercises, and meditation techniques.

Accessibility: Chair yoga is designed to make yoga accessible to people who may have mobility issues, balance problems, or difficulty getting up and down from the floor. It allows seniors to enjoy the benefits of yoga without the need for getting on the ground.

Adaptability: Chair yoga can be adapted to suit individual needs and abilities. It offers a variety of poses and movements that can be modified based on flexibility, strength, and range of motion.

Focus on Breath: Like traditional yoga, chair yoga emphasizes the importance of breath awareness and mindful breathing techniques. Participants are encouraged to synchronize breath with movement to promote relaxation and reduce stress.

B. Benefits of Chair Yoga for Seniors:

Improved Flexibility: Chair yoga helps seniors improve flexibility by gently stretching muscles and joints. This can lead to increased range of motion and easier movement in daily activities.

Enhanced Strength: Chair yoga includes strength-building exercises that target muscles throughout the body. Over time, these exercises can help seniors maintain or increase muscle mass and improve overall strength.

Better Balance and Stability: Many chair yoga poses focus on improving balance and stability, which can help reduce the risk of falls in seniors.

Stress Reduction: Chair yoga incorporates relaxation techniques such as deep breathing and guided meditation, which can help seniors reduce stress and anxiety.

Improved Posture: Practicing chair yoga can help seniors improve their posture by strengthening core muscles and promoting spinal alignment.

Enhanced Mind-Body Connection: Chair yoga encourages seniors to become more aware of their bodies and their breath, fostering a deeper connection between mind and body.

C. Overview of the Book's Structure:

Introduction: Provides an overview of chair yoga, its benefits, and why it's particularly beneficial for seniors.

Getting Started: Offers guidance on how to set up for chair yoga practice, including choosing a suitable chair and creating a comfortable environment.

Basic Poses and Movements: Introduces a series of beginner-friendly chair yoga poses and movements, with step-by-step instructions and illustrations.

Advanced Poses and Variations: Explores more challenging chair yoga poses and variations for seniors who want to deepen their practice.

Breathing Exercises and Meditation: Provides instructions for various breathing exercises and meditation techniques to promote relaxation and stress relief.

Safety Tips and Modifications: Offers safety tips and modifications for seniors with specific health concerns or physical limitations.

Sample Routines: Includes sample chair yoga routines that seniors can follow for a full-body workout or targeted practice.

Conclusion: Summarizes the key benefits of chair yoga for seniors and encourages readers to incorporate it into their daily routine for improved health and well-being.

UNDERSTANDING CHAIR YOGA

A. What is Chair Yoga?

Chair yoga is a form of yoga practice that modifies traditional yoga poses to be performed while sitting on a chair or using a chair for support. It is designed to make yoga accessible to individuals who may have mobility issues, balance problems, or difficulty getting up and down from the floor. Chair yoga incorporates gentle stretches, breathing exercises, and meditation techniques, offering a holistic approach to wellness that benefits both the body and mind.

B. History and Origin:

The precise origins of chair yoga are somewhat unclear, but it is believed to have emerged as a response to the need for more accessible forms of yoga practice. Some sources attribute the development of chair yoga to Lakshmi Voelker-Binder, a yoga instructor who began teaching chair yoga in the 1980s as a way to make yoga accessible to seniors and individuals with physical limitations. Since then, chair yoga has gained popularity and has been adapted and expanded by various yoga teachers and healthcare professionals to suit the needs of different populations.

C. How Chair Yoga Differs from Traditional Yoga:

Seated Poses: Chair yoga primarily consists of seated poses, whereas traditional yoga often involves standing, kneeling, and lying down poses.

Use of Props: Chair yoga typically incorporates the use of props such as chairs, blocks, and straps to support and modify poses, whereas traditional yoga may rely less on props.

Accessibility: Chair yoga is specifically designed to be accessible to individuals with limited mobility, balance issues, or other physical limitations, making it suitable for seniors and those with disabilities. Traditional yoga classes may not always address these specific needs.

Focus on Core and Stability: Chair yoga often emphasizes strengthening the core and improving stability, as many poses are performed while seated. Traditional yoga may focus more on flexibility and balance in standing or floor-based poses.

Adaptability: Chair yoga can be easily adapted to suit individual needs and abilities, with modifications available for almost every pose. Traditional yoga classes may offer modifications but may not always cater to the specific needs of seniors or individuals with physical limitations.

CHAPTER ONE

PHYSICAL BENEFITS OF CHAIR YOGA

A. Improving Flexibility

B. Enhancing Strength And Balance

C. Relieving Joint Pain And Tension

A. Improving Flexibility:

Gentle Stretching: Chair yoga incorporates gentle stretching movements that target muscles and joints throughout the body.

Increased Range of Motion: Regular practice of chair yoga can help improve flexibility by gradually increasing the range of motion in joints.

Reduced Stiffness: By encouraging movement in a safe and supported manner, chair yoga helps reduce stiffness in muscles and joints, promoting greater flexibility over time.

Enhanced Mobility: Improved flexibility enables seniors to perform daily activities with greater ease and comfort, such as bending, reaching, and twisting.

B. Enhancing Strength and Balance:

Muscle Engagement: Chair yoga incorporates strength-building exercises that target muscles in the arms, legs, core, and back.

Stability Challenges: Many chair yoga poses require seniors to engage their core muscles and maintain balance, which helps strengthen the muscles that support good posture and stability.

Reducing Falls Risk: By improving strength and balance, chair yoga can help reduce the risk of falls in seniors, enhancing overall safety and confidence in movement.

Functional Strength: Chair yoga exercises are designed to enhance functional strength, making it easier for seniors to perform everyday tasks such as standing up from a chair, walking, and climbing stairs.

C. Relieving Joint Pain and Tension:

Gentle Movement: Chair yoga promotes gentle movement of the joints, which can help reduce stiffness and alleviate discomfort associated with conditions such as arthritis.

Muscle Relaxation: Through relaxation techniques and mindful breathing, chair yoga helps release tension in muscles, relieving strain on the joints.

Improved Circulation: The flowing movements and deep breathing in chair yoga help improve circulation, which can reduce inflammation and promote healing in the joints.

Pain Management: Chair yoga can be an effective tool for managing chronic pain conditions by promoting relaxation, reducing muscle tension, and improving overall physical well-being.

CHAPTER TWO

MENTAL AND EMOTIONAL BENEFITS OF CHAIR YOGA

A. Reducing Stress And Anxiety

B. Improving Mood And Well-Being

C. Enhancing Mindfulness And Focus

A. Reducing Stress and Anxiety:

Deep Breathing: Chair yoga emphasizes deep, mindful breathing techniques, which activate the body's relaxation response and help reduce stress and anxiety.

Stress Relief: The gentle, flowing movements of chair yoga promote relaxation and calmness, helping to alleviate feelings of stress and tension in the body and mind.

Cortisol Regulation: Regular practice of chair yoga has been shown to help regulate cortisol levels, the stress hormone, leading to a more balanced and resilient response to stressors.

Emotional Regulation: Chair yoga encourages participants to cultivate self-awareness and emotional regulation skills, empowering them to manage stress and anxiety more effectively.

B. Improving Mood and Well-being:

Endorphin Release: Chair yoga stimulates the release of endorphins, the body's natural feel-good hormones, which can elevate mood and promote a sense of well-being.

Positive Affirmations: Many chair yoga classes incorporate positive affirmations and guided imagery, which can uplift mood and foster a positive outlook on life.

Social Connection: Participating in chair yoga classes provides an opportunity for social interaction and support, which can contribute to improved mood and emotional well-being.

Sense of Accomplishment: Chair yoga offers participants a sense of accomplishment and empowerment as they engage in gentle movement and self-care practices, boosting self-esteem and confidence.

C. Enhancing Mindfulness and Focus:

Mind-Body Connection: Chair yoga encourages participants to cultivate awareness of their breath, body sensations, and thoughts, fostering a deeper connection between mind and body.

Focused Attention: Chair yoga poses require concentration and focus on the present moment, helping to quiet the mind and reduce distractions.

Stress Reduction: By promoting mindfulness and present-moment awareness, chair yoga helps individuals let go of worries about the past or future, leading to reduced stress and increased relaxation.

Improved Cognitive Function: Regular practice of chair yoga has been linked to improvements in cognitive function, including attention, memory, and executive function, enhancing overall mental clarity and focus.

GETTING STARTED WITH CHAIR YOGA

A. Selecting The Right Chair

B. Creating A Safe And Comfortable Space

C. Warm-Up Exercises And Precautions

A. Selecting the Right Chair: Sturdy and Stable: Choose a chair that is sturdy and stable, with four solid legs and a flat seat. Avoid chairs with wheels or armrests that may move unexpectedly during practice.

Comfortable Seat: Select a chair with a comfortable seat cushion that provides adequate support without being too soft or too firm.

Proper Height: The chair should be at a height where your feet can rest comfortably flat on the floor, with knees bent at a 90-degree angle. If the chair is too tall, you can place yoga blocks or sturdy books under your feet for support.

Back Support: Look for a chair with good back support, preferably with a straight backrest that allows you to sit upright comfortably.

B. Creating a Safe and Comfortable Space:

Clearing the Area: Ensure that the space around your chair is clear of any obstacles or tripping hazards.

Non-Slip Surface: Practice chair yoga on a non-slip surface, such as a yoga mat or carpet, to prevent the chair from sliding during movement.

Adequate Lighting: Make sure the room is well-lit to prevent accidents and enhance visibility during practice.

Comfortable Temperature: Set the room temperature to a comfortable level to promote relaxation and prevent discomfort during practice.

Quiet Environment: Choose a quiet and peaceful environment for your chair yoga practice to minimize distractions and promote mindfulness.

C. Warm-Up Exercises and Precautions:

Gentle Movement: Begin your chair yoga practice with gentle warm-up exercises to prepare your body for movement. This may include shoulder rolls, neck stretches, and wrist circles.

Breathing Techniques: Practice deep breathing exercises to center your mind and connect with your breath before starting more dynamic movements.

Respect Your Body: Listen to your body and respect its limits. Avoid pushing yourself into discomfort or pain, and modify poses as needed to suit your individual needs and abilities.

Stay Hydrated: Drink water before, during, and after your chair yoga practice to stay hydrated and prevent dehydration.

Consult Your Healthcare Provider: If you have any existing health conditions or concerns, consult with your healthcare provider before starting a chair yoga practice to ensure that it is safe and appropriate for you.

CHAPTER THREE

CHAIR YOGA POSES AND SEQUENCES

A. Gentle Neck and Shoulder Stretches:

Neck Rolls: Sit tall in your chair with your feet flat on the floor. Slowly lower your chin towards your chest and begin to roll your head gently from side to side, allowing your ear to approach your shoulder. Repeat several times in each direction.

Shoulder Rolls: Sit upright and relax your shoulders. Inhale as you lift your shoulders up towards your ears, then exhale as you roll them back and down. Repeat this movement several times, alternating between forward and backward shoulder rolls.

Neck Stretch: Sit tall and reach your right arm down towards the floor, placing your palm on the seat of the chair. Gently tilt your head to the left, bringing your left ear towards your left shoulder until you feel a stretch along the right side of your neck. Hold for 15-30 seconds, then switch sides.

B. Seated Twists and Spinal Movements:

Seated Twist: Sit tall with your feet flat on the floor. Inhales as you lengthen your spine, then exhale as you twist to the right, placing your left hand on the outside of your right thigh and your right hand on the back of the chair. Hold the twist for a few breaths, then inhale back to center and repeat on the other side.

Seated Cat-Cow: Place your hands on your knees and sit tall. Inhale as you arch your back, lifting your chest and tilting your pelvis forward (Cow Pose). Exhale as you round your spine, tucking your chin towards your chest and pressing your hands into your knees (Cat Pose). Repeat this flowing movement with each breath for several rounds.

Forward Fold: Sit tall with your feet flat on the floor. Inhale as you lengthen your spine, then exhales as you hinge forward from your hips, reaching your hands towards your feet or the floor. Allow your head to relax and your spine to lengthen as you fold forward.

Hold for a few breaths, then slowly roll back up to a seated position.

C. Leg Stretches and Strengthening Exercises:

Seated Leg Extension: Sit tall with your feet flat on the floor. Extend your right leg straight out in front of you, flexing your foot. Hold for a few breaths, then lower your leg and repeat on the other side.

Chair Squats: Stand behind your chair and hold onto the back for support. Inhale as you bend your knees and lower your hips towards the chair, keeping your chest lifted and your weight in your heels. Exhale as you press through your heels to return to standing. Repeat for several reps.

Ankle Circles: Sit tall with your feet flat on the floor. Lift your right foot off the ground and begin to circle your ankle in one direction, then switch to the other direction. Repeat with your left foot.

CHAPTER FOUR

ADAPTING CHAIR YOGA FOR DIFFERENT NEEDS

A. Modifications For Limited Mobility

B. Yoga Props And Tools For Support

C. Incorporating Breathwork And Meditation

A. Modifications for Limited Mobility:

Seated Poses: Modify traditional standing poses to be performed while seated on a chair. For example, instead of a standing forward fold, perform a seated forward fold by sitting on the edge of the chair and folding forward from the hips.

Chair Support: Use the chair for support and stability during poses. For example, hold onto the backrest or sides of the chair during standing poses to help maintain balance.

Reduced Range of Motion: Adapt poses to accommodate limited range of motion in joints. For example, if reaching overhead is challenging, perform arm stretches at shoulder height or lower.

Chair Variations: Explore variations of poses that are specifically designed for seated practice, such as seated twists, leg lifts, and gentle backbends.

B. Yoga Props and Tools for Support:

Chair: Utilize the chair as a prop for support and stability during poses. For example, use the seat of the chair as a platform for seated poses and the backrest for support during standing poses.

Blocks: Place yoga blocks under the feet or hands to provide additional support and stability during poses. For example, use blocks under the hands in a seated forward fold to reduce strain on the lower back.

Straps: Use yoga straps to extend reach and facilitate movement in poses. For example, use a strap to hold onto the foot in a seated hamstring stretch if reaching the foot directly is not possible.

Blankets or Cushions: Place blankets or cushions on the seat of the chair or under the knees for added comfort and support during seated poses or kneeling positions.

C. Incorporating Breathwork and Meditation:

Deep Breathing: Integrate deep breathing exercises into chair yoga practice to promote relaxation and reduce stress. Encourage participants to focus on slow, rhythmic breathing patterns.

Guided Meditation: Lead guided meditation sessions focusing on relaxation, mindfulness, and inner peace. Use visualization techniques to help participants connect with their breath and cultivate a sense of calm.

Mindful Movement: Encourage participants to practice mindful movement by synchronizing breath with movement during chair yoga poses. Emphasize the importance of being present in the moment and paying attention to sensations in the body.

Body Scan: Guide participants through a body scan meditation to help them cultivate awareness of physical sensations and release tension in the body. Encourage participants to scan their body from head to toe, noticing areas of tension and consciously relaxing them.

CHAPTER FIVE

CHAIR YOGA ROUTINES FOR DAILY PRACTICE

A. Morning Wake-Up Routine

B. Afternoon Energy Boost

C. Evening Relaxation Sequence

A. Morning Wake-Up Routine: Seated Cat-Cow: Sit tall in your chair with your feet flat on the floor. Inhale as you arch your back (Cow Pose), lifting your chest and tilting your pelvis forward. Exhale as you round your spine (Cat Pose), tucking your chin towards your chest. Repeat for several rounds, flowing with your breath.

Neck Rolls: Gently roll your head from side to side, allowing your ear to approach your shoulder. Take slow, deep breaths as you release tension from the neck and shoulders.

Chair Forward Fold: Sit forward on the edge of your chair with your feet hip-width apart. Inhale as you lengthen your spine, then exhale as you hinge forward from your hips, reaching your hands towards your feet or the floor. Hold for a few breaths, then slowly roll back up to a seated position.

Seated Twist: Sit tall with your feet flat on the floor. Inhale as you lengthen your spine, then exhale as you twist to the right, placing your left hand on the outside of your right thigh and your right hand on the back of the chair. Hold for a few breaths, then inhale back to center and repeat on the other side.

Deep Breathing: Finish with a few rounds of deep breathing exercises, inhaling through the nose and exhaling through the mouth. Focus on filling your lungs with air and releasing tension with each exhale.

B. Afternoon Energy Boost:

Chair Sun Salutations: Begin seated with your hands together at heart center. Inhale as you reach your arms overhead, lifting your gaze towards the ceiling. Exhale as you bring your hands back to heart center. Repeat for several rounds, flowing with your breath.

Chair Warrior Poses: Sit tall with your feet flat on the floor. Inhale as you reach your arms overhead and lift your chest. Exhale as you twist to the right, placing your left hand on the outside of your right thigh and your right hand on the back of the chair. Hold for a few breaths, then inhale back to center and repeat on the other side.

Chair Leg Extensions: Sit tall with your feet flat on the floor. Inhale as you extend your right leg straight out in front of you, flexing your foot. Hold for a few breaths, then lower your leg and repeat on the other side. Alternate between legs for several rounds.

Chair Mountain Pose: Sit tall with your feet flat on the floor and your hands resting on your thighs. Close your eyes and take several deep breaths, grounding yourself into the present moment. Visualize yourself drawing energy up from the earth with each inhale and releasing tension with each exhale.

Chair Relaxation: Finish with a few minutes of seated relaxation, allowing your body to rest and recharge. Close your eyes, soften your breath, and let go of any tension or stress.

C. Evening Relaxation Sequence:
Seated Forward Fold: Sit forward on the edge of your chair with your feet hip-width apart. Inhale as you lengthen your spine, then exhale as you hinge

forward from your hips, reaching your hands towards your feet or the floor. Hold for a few breaths, then slowly roll back up to a seated position.

Chair Child's Pose: Sit tall with your knees bent and feet flat on the floor. Separate your knees slightly wider than hip-width apart and fold forward, resting your torso on your thighs and your forehead on the chair seat. Extend your arms forward or rest them by your sides. Take several deep breaths, allowing your body to relax and release tension.

Gentle Neck and Shoulder Stretches: Gently roll your head from side to side, releasing tension from the neck and shoulders. You can also reach your arms overhead and interlace your fingers, stretching upward and then leaning gently to one side to stretch the side body.

Chair Twist: Sit tall with your feet flat on the floor. Inhale as you lengthen your spine, then exhale as you twist to the right, placing your left hand on the outside of your right thigh and your right hand on the back of the chair. Hold for a few breaths, then inhale back to center and repeat on the other side.

Final Relaxation: Finish with a few minutes of seated relaxation, allowing your body and mind to unwind before bedtime. Close your eyes, soften your breath, and let go of any remaining tension or worries. Simply be present in the stillness and silence of the moment.

CHAPTER SIX

CHAIR YOGA FOR SPECIFIC HEALTH CONDITIONS

A. Arthritis And Joint Health

B. Osteoporosis And Bone Strength

C. Cardiovascular Health And Circulation

A. Arthritis and Joint Health:

Gentle Movements: Focus on gentle movements that promote flexibility and range of motion in the joints without exacerbating pain. Slow, controlled movements help to lubricate the joints and reduce stiffness.

Joint-Friendly Poses: Choose poses that are gentle on the joints, such as seated twists, gentle stretches, and slow, controlled movements. Avoid poses that involve deep or sudden movements that may strain the joints.

Use of Props: Utilize props like blankets, blocks, or cushions to provide support and cushioning for sensitive joints. For example, placing a folded blanket under the knees during kneeling poses can help reduce discomfort.

Warm-Up and Cool Down: Incorporate gentle warm-up exercises at the beginning of the session to prepare the joints for movement, and cool-down stretches at the end to promote relaxation and reduce tension.

Mindfulness and Breathing: Encourage participants to focus on their breath and practice mindfulness during chair yoga sessions. Deep breathing techniques can help reduce stress and tension, which may alleviate arthritis symptoms.

B. Osteoporosis and Bone Strength:

Weight-Bearing Poses: Include poses that promote bone strength and density, such as seated leg lifts, chair squats, and gentle standing poses with support from the chair. Weight-bearing exercises help stimulate bone growth and maintain bone density.

Spinal Extension: Incorporate poses that promote spinal extension and strengthen the back muscles, which can help improve posture and reduce the risk of fractures. Examples include seated backbends and gentle twists.

Balance Poses: Practice balance poses with the support of the chair to improve stability and reduce the risk of falls. Balancing poses help strengthen the muscles around the joints and improve coordination.

Safety and Alignment: Emphasize proper alignment and safe movement patterns to protect the spine and joints. Encourage participants to move mindfully and avoid sudden or jerky movements that may increase the risk of injury.

Gradual Progression: Start with gentle movements and gradually increase intensity and duration as participants become stronger and more confident. Encourage participants to listen to their bodies and modify poses as needed to suit their individual needs.

C. Cardiovascular Health and Circulation:

Dynamic Movements: Include dynamic movements that increase heart rate and improve circulation, such as seated marching, arm circles, and gentle twists. Dynamic movements help stimulate blood flow and promote cardiovascular health.

Breathwork: Integrate breathwork exercises that emphasize deep, diaphragmatic breathing. Slow, rhythmic breathing techniques help reduce stress, lower blood pressure, and improve oxygenation of the blood.

Chair Cardio: Incorporate cardiovascular exercises such as seated jumping jacks, seated jogging, or chair aerobics to increase heart rate and boost circulation. Modify exercises as needed to accommodate individual fitness levels and mobility.

Pacing and Rest: Encourage participants to pace themselves and take breaks as needed during the session. Monitor heart rate and breathing, and encourage participants to rest and hydrate as needed to prevent overexertion.

Cool Down and Relaxation: End the session with a gentle cool-down sequence and relaxation techniques to promote recovery and reduce stress on the cardiovascular system. Gentle stretches and deep breathing help promote relaxation and enhance overall well-being.

CHAPTER SEVEN

CHAIR YOGA FOR MINDFULNESS AND STRESS RELIEF

A. Guided Meditation Practices:

Body Scan Meditation: Guide participants through a body scan meditation, where they systematically focus their attention on different parts of the body, bringing awareness to sensations without judgment. Start from the toes and work your way up to the head, encouraging participants to notice any areas of tension or relaxation.

Visualization Meditation: Lead participants through a guided visualization meditation, where they imagine themselves in a peaceful and serene setting, such as a beach or forest. Encourage them to use all their senses to vividly imagine the sights, sounds, and smells of this calming environment.

Loving-Kindness Meditation: Guide participants through a loving-kindness meditation, where they cultivate feelings of compassion and kindness towards themselves and others. Encourage them to repeat phrases such as "May I be happy, may I be healthy, may I be at peace" while focusing on their breath.

Mindful Eating Meditation: Lead participants through a mindful eating meditation, where they slowly and deliberately eat a small piece of food, such as a raisin or a piece of chocolate, paying attention to the taste, texture, and sensations in their mouth. Encourage them to eat with full awareness and appreciation for each bite.

Body Awareness Meditation: Guide participants through a body awareness meditation, where they bring attention to the sensations in their body as they breathe. Encourage them to notice the rise and fall of their chest, the feeling of air entering and leaving their nostrils, and any other physical sensations that arise.

B. Deep Breathing Techniques:
Diaphragmatic Breathing: Teach participants how to engage in diaphragmatic breathing, where they breathe deeply into their belly rather than shallowly into their chest.

Encourage them to place one hand on their abdomen and the other hand on their chest, and to focus on making their belly rise and fall with each breath.

4-7-8 Breathing: Teach participants the 4-7-8 breathing technique, where they inhale for a count of 4, hold their breath for a count of 7, and exhale for a count of 8. Encourage them to repeat this pattern several times, focusing on the rhythm of their breath and the sensation of relaxation with each exhale.

Alternate Nostril Breathing: Guide participants through alternate nostril breathing, where they use their fingers to gently close one nostril while inhaling and exhaling through the other nostril. Encourage them to switch nostrils and continue this pattern, noticing the balancing and calming effect on their mind and body.

Square Breathing: Teach participants square breathing, where they inhale for a count of 4, hold their breath for a count of 4, exhale for a count of 4, and then hold their breath again for a count of 4 before starting the cycle again. Encourage them to visualize the shape of a square as they breathe, focusing on each side of the square.

Ocean Breathing: Guide participants through ocean breathing, where they imagine themselves lying on a beach and listening to the sound of ocean waves. Encourage them to inhale deeply through their nose, imagining the sound of the waves crashing onto the shore, and exhale slowly and audibly through their mouth, imagining the sound of the waves receding back into the ocean.

C. Cultivating Gratitude and Presence:

Gratitude Journaling: Encourage participants to keep a gratitude journal, where they write down three things they are grateful for each day. This practice helps cultivate a sense of appreciation and abundance, shifting focus away from stressors and towards positive aspects of life.

Mindful Walking: Guide participants through a mindful walking meditation, where they take slow, deliberate steps and pay attention to the sensations in their feet as they make contact with the ground. Encourage them to notice the sights, sounds, and smells around them as they walk, bringing full awareness to the present moment.

Mindful Movement: Lead participants through a series of mindful movement exercises, such as gentle stretches or yoga poses, focusing on the sensations in their body and the rhythm of their breath. Encourage them to move slowly and intentionally, staying fully present with each movement.

Gratitude Circle: Create a gratitude circle where participants take turns expressing something they are grateful for. This practice fosters a sense of connection and community, as well as a deeper appreciation for the blessings in life.

Sensory Awareness: Guide participants through a sensory awareness exercise, where they bring attention to each of their five senses one at a time. Encourage them to notice the sights, sounds, smells, tastes, and textures around them, fully immersing themselves in the present moment.

CHAIR YOGA FOR OVERALL WELL-BEING

A. Lifestyle Tips for Healthy Aging:

Stay Active: Incorporate regular physical activity into your routine, including chair yoga, walking, swimming, or other low-impact exercises. Aim for at least 30 minutes of activity most days of the week to support mobility, flexibility, and cardiovascular health.

Eat Well: Maintain a balanced diet rich in fruits, vegetables, lean proteins, whole grains, and healthy fats. Stay hydrated and limits processed foods, sugary snacks, and excessive alcohol consumption to support overall health and vitality.

Prioritize Sleep: Aim for 7-9 hours of quality sleep each night to support physical and mental health. Establish a regular sleep schedule, create a relaxing bedtime routine, and create a comfortable sleep environment to promote restful sleep.

Manage Stress: Practice stress management techniques such as deep breathing, mindfulness, meditation, or relaxation exercises to reduce stress and promote emotional well-being. Prioritize self-care activities that bring you joy and relaxation.

Stay Socially Connected: Maintain relationships with friends, family, and community members to foster social connection and support. Participate in social activities, clubs, or volunteer opportunities to stay engaged and connected with others.

B. Integrating Chair Yoga into Daily Life:

Set Realistic Goals: Start with small, achievable goals for integrating chair yoga into your daily routine, such as practicing for 10-15 minutes each day or attending a weekly chair yoga class.

Create a Dedicated Space: Designate a quiet, comfortable space in your home for practicing chair yoga. Set up a chair, yoga mat, and any props you may need to support your practice.

Schedule Regular Practice Times: Establish a consistent schedule for practicing chair yoga, whether it's in the morning, during a break at work, or in the evening before bed. Consistency is key to establishing a sustainable practice.

Be Flexible and Adaptive: Be open to adapting your chair yoga practice to fit your schedule and lifestyle. If you're short on time, try incorporating shorter practice sessions or practicing chair yoga poses throughout the day.

Incorporate Mindful Moments: Look for opportunities to incorporate mindfulness and relaxation techniques into your daily activities, such as deep breathing exercises during stressful moments or mindful walking during a break at work.

C. Long-Term Benefits and Sustainability:

Physical Health: Regular practice of chair yoga can lead to improved flexibility, strength, balance, and range of motion, which can help support overall physical health and mobility as you age.

Emotional Well-being: Chair yoga promotes relaxation, stress reduction, and emotional balance, leading to improved mental health and well-being over time.

Social Connection: Participating in chair yoga classes or group sessions provides an opportunity for social interaction and support, fostering a sense of community and belonging.

Cognitive Health: Chair yoga incorporates mindfulness and cognitive engagement, which can help support cognitive function and brain health as you age.

Sustainability: Chair yoga is a sustainable form of exercise that can be practiced safely and comfortably throughout the lifespan. It can be adapted to suit individual needs and

abilities, making it accessible to people
of all ages and fitness levels.

CONCLUSION

A. Recap of Chair Yoga's Benefits: Chair yoga offers a wide range of benefits for physical, mental, and emotional well-being.

It improves flexibility, strength, balance, and range of motion, making it accessible to people of all ages and fitness levels.

Chair yoga promotes relaxation, stress reduction, and emotional balance, fostering a sense of peace and calm.

It can help manage chronic conditions such as arthritis, osteoporosis, and cardiovascular issues, providing gentle and effective exercise.

Chair yoga enhances mindfulness, cognitive function, and overall quality of life, supporting healthy aging and vitality.

B. Encouragement for Continued Practice:

I encourage you to continue incorporating chair yoga into your daily routine to reap its many benefits.

Even a few minutes of chair yoga each day can make a significant difference in your physical and mental well-being.

Remember to listen to your body, honor your limitations, and practice self-compassion as you embark on your chair yoga journey.

Stay committed to your practice and be patient with yourself as you progress and grow in your yoga practice.

C. Resources for Further Exploration and Support:

Consider attending chair yoga classes at your local yoga studio, community center, or senior center to deepen your practice and connect with others.

Explore online resources such as videos, articles, and books on chair yoga to expand your knowledge and discover new techniques.

Connect with certified chair yoga instructors or yoga therapists for personalized guidance and support tailored to your specific needs and goals.

Join online forums, social media groups, or support networks dedicated to chair yoga and healthy aging to connect with like-minded individuals and share experiences.

THE END

www.ingramcontent.com/pod-product-compliance
Lightning Source LLC
Chambersburg PA
CBHW061255250726

48653CB00002B/665